Ketogenic Diet

The Real Truth -

Ketogenic Recipes for Weight Loss

Jim Berry

Disclaimer

The information contained in this book is strictly for educational purpose only. The content of this book is the sole expression and opinion of its author and not necessarily that of the publisher. It is not intended to cure, treat, and diagnose any kind of disease or medical condition. It is sold with the understanding that the publisher is not rendering any type of medical, psychological, legal, or any other kind of professional advice. You should seek the services of a competent professional before applying concepts in this book. Neither the publisher nor the individual author(s) shall be liable for any physical, psychological, emotional, financial, or commercial damages, directly or indirectly by the use of this material, which is provided "as is", and without warranties. Therefore, if you wish to apply ideas contained in this book, you are taking full responsibility for your actions.

Table of Contents

Introduction

Ketogenic diet is a type of dieting program developed to promote the state of "ketosis", which aids in weight loss by making the body burn body fats rather than carbohydrates. This diet has created a breakthrough due to its proven effectiveness. However, it must be noted that the rate of weight loss depends on several factors, such as your metabolism rate and the amount of fat you want to get rid of.

In this diet, you are allowed to consume a low carbohydrate diet, moderate protein and high-fat diet in order to put your body into ketosis. Most people refer to it as the low-carb diet due to its nature.

By eating fewer carbs, the ketone levels in the body are heightened. Anyone who is into ketogenic diet must achieve ketosis for the diet to take effect.

Basically, the ketogenic works only if the body gets into the state of ketosis. How does this take place?

Well, the body depends on glucose as its main fuel - glucose is produced by the break-down of carbohydrates and transformed into energy which the body uses to power the organs and muscles. When the intake of carbs is limited, there will be a shortage in glucose. When this happens, the liver will produce ketones which make the burns body fats for fuel instead. Thus, there will be a quick reduction in weight and body fats.

It must be noted that ketones are acidic compounds and may lead to serious problems. If ketone levels are neglected, you may suffer from heightened blood acidity and other problems related to kidney and the liver. Yet, when used properly and with full responsibility, this diet can not only help you lose weight but it will have many beneficial effects to your health.

Not only does ketogenic diet help in dealing with excessive weight and obesity, it is treated in epilepsy. The diet has also been found to have good effects in cardiovascular diseases as well as type 2 diabetes.

On an average, the body can attain desirable ketone levels for weight loss and other conditions within a period of 2-4 weeks. Any person on a ketogenic diet should maintain a certain ketone level, which is at 0.5 to 3mmol/L. But then, some people do not experience any problems even if their ketone levels are at 5mmol/L.

Measuring the amount of ketones in your body is very easy. You may use a urine dipstick kit, which is both affordable and reliable method. There are also the blood test kits, but these are a bit more expensive.

1: Pros and Cons

Every diet program has its ups and downs, so does the ketogenic diet. However, despite the many controversies that surrounds it, the positive points of the diet outweighs the negative ones based on the great number of studies conducted on low carb or ketogenic diets.

Pros

There are a lot of good things to expect during the first few months after making a shift to the ketogenic diet.

It reduces appetite

This is one of the main reasons why people lose weight when on the ketogenic diet. It suppresses the appetite - but in a healthy way!

Strong appetite is what makes people horrible when dieting.

Controlling the appetite is among the hardest things to do, especially if you love food. I bet you know knew that! But the good news is ketogenic diet actually makes you consume less food and fewer calories.

With high fat and protein consumption, there will be less hunger as the ketones fight your appetite. In fact, you may forget to eat at times and this fact can appeal to you if you are the kind of person who struggles with food cravings.

More weight loss

Do you know that trimming your carb intake is one of the best strategies to get rid of unwanted body fats? So, why avoid healthy fats in foods?

According to research, individuals who are on the ketogenic diet tend to lose more weight than those who consumes less fat. This is because ketogenic diet expels excess water out of the body. With reduced levels of insulin, the kidney releases extra sodium resulting to fast weight loss, which may occur as early as the first week.

But then, you need to stick to this diet in order to gain long term benefits.

Lowers cholesterol levels

Cholesterol is produced by surplus glucose in the body. By consuming less glucose, you are actually doing your body a favor as it results in lower cholesterol levels. This drop in the level of cholesterol will also reduce the damage to the arteries and the heart.

In relation to this, ketogenic diet can elevate HDL or high-density lipoprotein levels known as the good cholesterol while lowering the LDL or low-density lipoprotein called as the bad cholesterol. This benefit also targets those who are suffering from heart diseases, particularly hypertension. With lower cholesterol levels, high blood pressure is prevented leading to a healthier and longer life along with a reduced incidence of developing other types of diseases.

Fat loss in the tummy area

Excessive bulk of fat in the tummy is not only unpleasant, but could also lead to insulin resistance as well as metabolic dysfunction. The great thing with a low carb diet is that it promotes weight loss in the abdominal area. Hence, the ketogenic diet is proven to be effective if you are trying to eliminate those belly bags.

Over a long period of use, this diet could also reduce the risk for diabetes type 2 and a number of heart diseases.

Better digestion

With this low carb diet, your digestive system will improve significantly. After a few weeks after the shift, you will feel a reduced incidence of gas pains, bloating, tummy pains and other symptoms of poor digestion. All of these are due to the reduced consumption of glucose.

Less joint pain/stiffness and heartburn

The ketogenic diet reduces carbs and grainy foods from your regular diet. Grains are one of the major culprits in muscle pains and joint stiffness. By not eating fewer grains, there will be reduced pains.

Another condition relieved by eating fewer grains and sugar is heartburn. Hence, the ketogenic diet does not only aid in weight loss, but also in various health conditions.

Improved mood control

Ketones are found to be highly beneficial in making the neurotransmitters in the body, like dopamine and serotonin more controllable. The end result is mood stabilization.

Cons

There are few side effects associated with the ketogenic diet, but these can be minimized when you are aware of the symptoms and why they happen. Plus, these side effects diminish after several weeks when your body has adjusted to the ketones.

For your best knowledge, here are the most common side effects:

Headache

This is just a normal thing as your body adapts to the state of ketosis. This is usually brought by mineral deficiency as you cut down on carbohydrates and you expel high amounts of sodium. This symptom will subside in a matter 2-3 days, so there is nothing to worry about.

Frequent bathroom trips

You will be urinating a lot when you are on this low-carb diet. This is because your kidney is dumping the extra water released by the breakdown of glucose in your muscles and liver. However, the frequency of urination will reduce as your body gets used to ketosis and your carbohydrate intake goes down.

Constipation

Constipation is another side effect since the body is losing water and salt. This may also be brought by too many nuts and dairy in the diet. The best way to deal with this is to reduce the consumption of food that results in the condition and drink lots of water.

Weakness and dizziness

Expelling excess water in the body when in the ketogenic diet will also result in mineral loss - potassium, magnesium and sodium. This leaves you tired and a bit dizzy. To ease these symptoms, all you need to do is to replace the minerals by taking mineral supplements or consume food high in minerals. For instance, banana and cantaloupe is rich in potassium. You may also take some broth since it could replenish sodium in your body.

Low blood sugar

Starting on a ketogenic may cause a drop in blood sugar, up to the point that you are suffering from "hypoglycemia". This is especially true if your body was used to a diet high in carbohydrates.

A sudden drop in the intake of carbs may confuse the insulin in the body - high insulin is produced on a high-carb diet. Hence, there can be episodes of hypoglycemia, which is manifested by cold clammy skin, excessive sweating, irritability, shakiness extreme hunger and palpitations.

The best remedy is to drink a glass of orange juice or take hard-sugared candy. So far, this is the scariest side effect of the ketogenic diet, so anyone who wishes to go on a diet should be careful. Also, consult a doctor before you start this diet.

2: Ketogenic Diet Basics

The ketogenic diet program is very simple - low carbohydrate diet, which allows you to consume real food. If you are the type of person who has been used to eating a diet rich in carbohydrates, or perhaps you are one of those fat phobic dieters out there, well you will really benefit a lot from this section.

In the ketogenic diet, you need to be a bit more specific about the amount of carbs, proteins and fats that you eat as well as your caloric intake. So, before anything else, take a look at these:

- Carbohydrates: A gram of carbohydrate is equivalent to 4 calories
- Proteins: A gram of protein is equivalent to 4 calories
- Fats: A gram of fat is equivalent to 9 calories

Now, the question is how much you should consume? Well, basically, simply stick to 10% calories coming from carbs, 30% from protein and 60% from fats.

However, you should not rush things as your body may not be able to compensate for the change. The best thing that you can do is to trim down your carb intake by 50% and then go lower after a few days until you reach the target limit that helps your body maintain ketosis. If your allowable carb intake is low, make sure you avoid fruits and carb loaded treats.

Stay moderate on your protein intake - ideally you should consume 1 to 2 grams of protein per 1 kilogram of body weight. If you weigh 50 kg, you should be eating about 50 to 100 grams of protein.

While, 60% of your diet should be composed of fats - don't feel bad, because you need lots of fats to keep your body in ketosis. After all, these fats get burned during the process. However, you should consume healthy fats, like omega 3s saturated and monounsaturated ones.

Unlike other diets, you do not have to control the amount of food that you eat in a deliberate manner. But then, you should know when to

stop when your tummy is already full, even when there is still food on your plate. The simplest rule is: just eat when you feel hungry and never let other people influence you on how frequent or what you eat.

Also, there is no need to strictly count your calorie intake while trying to lose weight using this diet. But you need to watch out for calories when you already achieved your weight goal. Of course, your body needs to adjust according to its needs.

Another thing that you should remember is to drink lots of water - as much as possible drink 2 to 3 liters per day.

You can't simply jump into the ketogenic diet without knowing about the essentials. This low carb diet thing is very simple, yet there are still measures that you need to observe. Before you begin dieting, here are a few things that you should bear in mind:

Take care of your electrolytes

The three macronutrients, such as carbs, proteins and fat are not the only areas that you should look into as vitamins, minerals as well as electrolytes in the body are important as well.

Electrolytes, such as potassium, sodium and magnesium are often excreted excessively when under the ketogenic diet - particularly if you are consuming less than 20g of carbohydrates.

To replenish the potassium in your body, you may take cantaloupes, mushroom and avocado and fish, like salmon. Or, simply mix a pinch of salt in a liter of water - the same thing to do with sodium deficiency. If you lack magnesium, consume a handful of nuts each day or take magnesium supplements. Make sure you do not exceed the recommended daily allowance!

Don't rely too much on low-carb products

Make it a habit to stick to unprocessed food and be aware of deceptive labeling. There are a lot of products labeled as "low carbs", but more often than that, these products have higher carb content than stated in the label. Also, stay away from aspartame and other artificial additives and flavorings as these can have detrimental effects not only on your body weight, but your overall health as well.

Basically, you should avoid anything that is low carb or fat-free as these food items usually have additives and not satiating at all making you hungry more often, so your cravings can be triggered too.

Always plan ahead

You should make an effort to plan in advance to help you get a good start with the ketogenic diet. The first step that you should take is to eliminate everything that is not allowed in the diet, such as sugary foods, sugar, flour and processed foods, among others. In short, get rid of anything that is tempting.

To avoid temptations, you should have a plan or have a list of foods to buy and meals to prepare for the whole week ahead. Don't go food shopping without something planned in mind as this will lead you to buying and eating foods that are not suitable for the ketogenic diet.

Carbs

There are many recommendations on how much you need to limit your carbohydrates in order to reach ketosis. Some suggest that all you need to do is lower your carbohydrate intake to less than 50 grams, some will even tell you that 100 grams or less is fine.

But the truth is that no one knows for sure because it varies from person to person. No two people are the same. We all have different levels of carbohydrate tolerance. The vast majority will need to keep their carbs under 50 grams, usually around 30 grams, but ultimately you will have to determine this for yourself by testing.

Your best bet is to start at about 40 grams of total carbs daily and adjust from there. After two weeks, if you are not producing enough ketones (below you'll learn how to measure them), slowly reduce your carbs by 5 grams a week until you do.

Protein intake

Despite what you may have heard, the ketogenic diet is NOT a high protein diet. In fact, eating too much protein can be a problem for some people, especially for those who are already sensitive to carbohydrates.

The problem with proteins is that your body, being the incredibly efficient machine that it is, has the ability to turn proteins into glucose (known as gluconeogenesis). Too much glucose can raise your insulin levels, preventing your body's ability to release and burn the fatty acids which leads to ketosis.

The amount of protein that causes gluconeogenesis varies from person to person, and depends on how insulin resistant you are.

To be safe, keep your protein consumption moderate at about .80 to 1.0 grams per each pound of lean body weight (depending on your activity level). If you work out and lift weights 3 times a week, use the higher number.

For example, if your lean body mass is 150 lbs.:

150 lbs. x .80 grams of protein =120 grams of protein per day or

150 lbs. x 1.0 grams protein =150 grams of protein per day

Calorie counting

Some will argue that calorie counting is not really necessary on a ketogenic diet, but if your goal is to lose weight then the law of thermogenic still applies.

Although many people report that they have successfully lost weight without counting calories, it's probably due to the fact that people did not eat as much because the ketogenic diet is very satisfying. And also because they did not have to deal with the constant insulin spikes caused by carbohydrates, they were not as hungry and were not tempted to cheat. Ketones also dampens your appetite.

However, we still recommend you start out with a moderate calorie deficit. Severely cutting back your calories is never a good idea and will usually backfire on you in the long run, causing metabolic damage.

Start with a calorie deficit of no more than 15-20% below maintenance levels. You can get a close approximation of your maintenance calories by multiplying your current weight by 15 or 16. Then multiply that number by .80 (80%) to give you a 20% deficit.

Example using the values for maintenance calories from the last section:

Female at 150 lbs. x 15 cal/lb. = 2250 cal/day.

A 20% deficit is 2250 x 0.80 = 1800

1800 calories/day

Male at 180 lbs. x 16 cal/lb. = 2880 cal/day

A 15% deficit is 2880 cal/day x 0.85 = 2448

2448 calories/day

These figures should be considered starting points only as they are based on averages and estimations for maintenance calorie levels. Some individuals may need to reduce calories further.

How are ketones measured?

Ketones are only produced when the insulin levels are low. A sure sign of low insulin is a high amount of ketones in the bloodstream. When your ketones are high, it is referred to as optimal ketosis.

So how do you know whether or not you have a healthy amount of ketones in your bloodstream?

The traditional way of checking is through a urine sample using urine test sticks (ketosis). They are the easiest to start with and you can buy them at any drugstore.

However, the longer you stay in ketosis, the less reliable urine sticks become because the kidneys become more efficient at absorbing ketones and fewer will show up in your urine. You may end up mistakenly thinking that ketosis is slowing down when in fact your body has just adapted to using ketones as its main energy source.

If you want a more accurate measure, there are many test gadgets that will test your blood for ketones that are now available for home use. They are reasonably priced as well.

It is ideal to measure your blood ketones in the morning on an empty stomach. If your blood ketone test result is at 1.5 to 3.0mmol/L, you are in an optimal ketosis, which means your body has reached a level ideal for maximum weight loss.

This is what you should be aiming for if you want to stop stalling and get over a weight loss plateau. Anything below or above these values is not recommended. That would mean you are still either getting a little more carbs or not getting an adequate amount of food.

For instance, blood ketones of 0.5mmol/L or below are not a ketosis level. At this point, you are not losing or burning fat. If your blood ketone is between 0.5 and 1.5mmol/L, you may be losing weight but you can do better. This is considered a light nutritional ketosis. It is ideal for fat burning but not an optimal one.

On the other hand, if your blood ketone level is above 3.0mmol/L then you've officially gone overboard and it's no longer healthy.

Additional reminders

- The list of things to observe when under the ketogenic diet is almost endless. To further guide you as you start on this dieting program, take a look at these:
- Eat meat, eggs and vegetables without much starch - these are good for you!
- Snack on nuts, like almonds and macadamia as well as fruits, like avocados.
- Don't be fat phobic! Use lard, coconut oil and palm oil with your cooking.
- When eating salad, grab some sesame oil, olive oil or anything organic.
- Avoid trans-fats as well as processed oils like margarine and hydrogenated oil.

3: Weight Loss

If you're interested in losing weight, then you should know the magic number for weight loss: to lose a pound of mass, you have to burn 3,500 more calories than you take in.

However, if you look around, not everyone appears to be carrying their weight the same way. Some of this comes from genetics, and some of this comes from lifestyle choices. Some people have a body type that amasses fat in the belly area, while others take fat more uniformly across their body.

While you can't fight your genes, you can make the right lifestyle choices when it comes to the fat that you take in, and starting a ketogenic diet will be one of the best choices you can make when it comes to removing your belly fat quickly. It is important to realize that hormones tell our body what to do with the food that comes in.

One of the most important hormones in this area is insulin. When you take in glucose, your body releases insulin, and any carbohydrates that you consume will break down into glucose. The more glucose you have in your bloodstream, the more insulin your body sets loose. Your body has to deal with glucose because if the levels get too high, glucose becomes a toxin.

As a result, your liver and muscles can store it, or your body can burn it through metabolic processes, or you can store it as fat. Because you're converting your body to ketosis, though, you won't burn glucose - but fat instead.

You're going to bring your carb consumption down close to zero, which means that the insulin hormone won't be circulating through your blood telling your body to shove fat into a place you don't want it. Instead, you'll be burning it.

This is why the ketogenic diet is one of the best ways to shed belly fat. Any low carb diet limits the glucose you're taking in, keeping you from spiking in glucose (and then spiking in insulin, and then storing glucose as fat).

A recent discovery of how insulin works makes it simple to understand why so many people in the West have issues with weight. So many meals have more than 100 grams of carbohydrates that digest quickly and then absorb as fat.

Pizza, sandwich bread, hamburger buns, noodles, cereals, and drinks with sugar all tell your body to send insulin around the body. These foods all contain processed carbohydrates. Because the body has an easier time breaking these down, the glucose inside hits our bloodstream more quickly and in greater volume than fruits and vegetables - even the starchy and sugary ones.

If you drink 20 ounce bottles of Coke or Sprite, you are taking in as much sugar as you would by eating nine cups of strawberries. Remember, glucose is ultimately toxic if the levels get too high. Your body, then, has to figure out what to do with it.

When you exercise you use the glucose that is in your muscles and the liver. If those areas have little or no glucose left, what you take in goes to those repositories before it goes to fat.

The average active person only needs 150 grams of carbohydrates each day to keep full levels of glycogen in the liver and muscles. In the West, the average person takes in about 300 grams of carbohydrates on a daily basis. Their activity levels are low (no, Facebooking doesn't count as exercise).

This means that each meal adds more glucose into your fat storage area. Also, every meal is followed by the introduction of a hormone (insulin) that hinders you from burning fat as energy. Wonder why it's so hard to lose weight?

You may also have read about the increasing number of cases of type 2 diabetes among Western societies. This increase is a direct consequence of the ways our diet influences our insulin. If you have been habitually eating a high carb diet, it is most likely you built up some degree of insulin resistance. You feel lethargic; you've gain weight, and you are at risk of type 2 diabetes. The good news is that you can turn this around by staying on the ketogenic diet.

Another hormone that you need to know when you are thinking about burning belly body fat is Cortisol. This is the hormone that your body uses to signal the need to release the energy that is being stored inside fat cells.

Your Cortisol levels are at their highest first thing in the morning. Any time your body has physical or mental stress, Cortisol enters the system as well. So a balanced Cortisol levels are a good thing.

However, because stress is part of our daily lives, it is easy for Cortisol levels to get out of control. When your Cortisol levels are too high, your body will fight fat loss and you will gain more weight. If there is a layer of fat on your belly that you just cannot get rid of no matter how hard you exercise, or how well you diet, your Cortisol levels are probably too high.

So how does the ketogenic diet interact with these hormones? The magic word here is leptin. This is the hormone that tells you to stop eating because you are full. Your body sends out a lot of leptin when you take in proteins and fats and sends out little when you take in carbohydrates.

Think about it. Would you be able to eat more slices of bacon or French toast sticks? Which would make you feel full (or even a little green at the gills) faster? The bacon will make you feel full sooner, and you'll feel full longer.

This is why so many healthy snacks for weight loss have protein in them, because they signal your body to send out leptin so you don't go back to the pantry for chips after you have your snack. Staying away from carbs and sticking with high protein and high fat meals, you stop eating sooner, your blood glucose levels stay manageable, and that belly fat starts to fall away, particularly if you stick with a regular exercise regimen.

4: Anti-Aging

When it comes to the aging process, there are quite a few theories going around. Some have to do with genetics, while others focus on the damage that takes place in body tissues and cellular structures. Having the knowledge of some of these theories can make the benefits of ketogenic diet easier to understand.

Free radicals and aging

The role of free radicals in aging is the basis of one of the most commonly promulgated aging theory. On just about every wellness website, you can come across these little things called "free radicals" as well as the solution for them, known as antioxidants.

Free radicals are molecules which are chemically reactive and they are commonly known as reactive oxygen species, or ROS. These connect to cells, leading to inflammation and damage to proteins and genetic material in the cell's nucleus.

These free radicals are called "chemically reactive" because they are short on electrons. They rove through cells looking for an electron to swipe from another molecule. The process through which this takes place is known as oxidation and it can lead to a sequence of damages.

When one electron gets stolen by a free radical, the victim molecule now is missing an electron, meaning that it is reactive too. It grabs an electron, and the vicious cycle continues. As time goes by, the damage increases and the aging process speeds up.

According to this theory, the best way to stop this sort of damage and retard the process of aging is to boost the level of antioxidants in the body. Antioxidants work because they have an electron to give away. They neutralize the free radicals by stopping the chain of damage before they can get started.

The majority of the free radicals in the body come from normal chemical reactions, like those that make energy inside our mitochondria. Other sources come from consuming a lot of polyunsaturated vegetable oils or smoking. Not having enough antioxidants leads to an increased level of damage. This is why increasing antioxidant level is so important in reversing the aging process.

Glycation and aging

The theory behind high blood sugars causing the aging process to accelerate centers around a process known as glycation. This involves excess glucose in the bloodstream binding to proteins that form the basis of our body tissues and cells.

As time goes by, these tissues form structures known as advanced glycation end products, or AGEs. These limit the efficiency of protein functions, to the point where proteins can no longer communicate or perform as necessary.

Such effects as atherosclerosis, nerve damage and vision loss, as well as complications associated with diabetes, are among the possibilities. Imagine pouring the syrup from a jar of maraschino cherries to your television remote; how can you expect the remote control to perform its normal functions?

As blood sugar levels go up, so does the glycation level. High fructose consumption appears to accelerate the process further - perhaps as much as 10 times when compared to simple glucose in the blood.

How ketogenic diet inhibit the aging process

There are several ways in which ketogenic diets inhibit the aging process. First, ketogenic diet cuts down baseline sugar levels in the blood. In simple terms, this cuts down the glycation rate, meaning that those advanced glycation end products do not form as quickly. The damage to your proteins, then, takes much longer to occur.

Ketogenic diet also reduces your triglycerides, fatty acids that show up in the bloodstream. This might seem counterintuitive because you are consuming more fats with this diet.

However, your body is learning to use the fat as fuel. Your fatty acids are being consumed by your body instead of being sent to your bloodstream. When your triglyceride count is high, your body has the tendency to produce more advanced glycation end products.

When your body enters ketosis, you produce more mitochondrial glutathione. This is a crucial antioxidant that operates inside your mitochondria, which is a main staging ground for the work of free radicals. One reason why this is so important is that many antioxidants that you consume orally have a hard time making it into the mitochondria, leaving the free radicals to do a great deal of damage.

Ketogenic diet boosts your body's creation of uric acid and other powerful natural antioxidants. One reason why this is so important, whether you're talking about aging, neurological protection or weight loss, the stress that oxidants provide wreaks havoc in matters from the brain to many of the cells throughout the body.

Conditions like ALS, Parkinson's disease, Alzheimer's disease, stroke and traumatic brain injury all appear to feature oxidative stress as a potential cause.

Finally, ketogenic diets improve your body's ability to manage blood sugar levels and curb hunger. When you're eating less, you're cutting down on the oxidative damage that takes place inside your body, according to a number of research studies.

So how does a ketogenic diet help stop the aging process? Based on existing research, there is a mechanism system in the body that appears to respond in a positive way to the changes that take place when the body enters ketosis by burning fats for energy instead of glucose.

When your blood sugar levels go down, so does the number of glycation, insulin levels in the blood, and inflammation. These three elements are closely connected with a wide variety of diseases that all contribute to earlier mortality.

In the final analysis, a ketogenic diet is a great way to cut your levels of insulin and blood sugar which will increase your sense of well-being as well as your longevity.

While there are some side effects that may show up in a small percentage of the people who switch to this diet, current research indicates that, for most people, the side effects are manageable and do not outweigh the benefits of weight loss and a slower aging process.

5: Brain Health

It's important to remember that the ketogenic diet actually creates a sensation of starvation, as the body changes over to the metabolic state known as ketosis. Instead of running on sugar, the body runs on fat -specifically, the ketone bodies your liver pulls out of fatty acids.

The three types of ketones are acetone, acetoacetate and BHB (beta hydroxybutyrate). When they enter the bloodstream, your brain and other organs snap them up and pull them into their mitochondria, using them for fuel. Extra ketones go out through your urine (although acetone comes out through your breath).

When your brain pulls these ketones in, it protects your brain from diseases. So while this diet came about as a way to manage epilepsy, it has also shown promise as a way to shield the brain in several other ways.

So how does this work? One possible answer has to do with energy. Many neurological disorders share one commonality: insufficient production of energy. When metabolic stress occurs, ketones provide another source of energy to keep normal metabolism in brain cells up and running.

It appears that BHB may be more efficient than glucose, giving more energy for each unit of oxygen in use. Ketogenic diets also boost the numbers of mitochondria, known as the brain's energy factories. One recent study located an enhanced gene expression when it comes to encoding for energy metabolism within your hippocampus (the brain sector dedicated to memory and learning) as well as mitochondrial enzymes.

When brain diseases related to age strikes, the cells in the hippocampus often degenerate. This leads to memory loss and cognitive issues. With a boost in the reserve energy, neurons may gain the ability to fight of the stressors that normally kill these cells.

Another possible benefit of the ketogenic diet for the brain is that this eating plan may reduce the effects of one of the prime sources of stress on neurons. When cellular metabolism takes place, reactive oxygen is one of the by-products. This is not the same thing as the oxygen we breathe; instead, these oxidants just have one electron.

As a result, they are more highly reactive, crashing into membranes and proteins. The more oxidants you have the more your risk of getting a stroke, neural degeneration, and the increased signs of aging. When you take in ketones, your body makes fewer of these oxidants and fights the ones that are already there.

Basically, a ketogenic diet acts like consuming berries on a large scale. Ketones boosts the work of glutathione peroxidase, which is part of our built in system that fights oxidants. Reducing carbohydrate intake also leads to reduced oxidation of glucose (called glycolysis).

Because the ketogenic diet is high in fat, it also boosts the polyunsaturated fatty acid levels in the body. Known as PUFAs, these also limit the production of oxidation as well as inflammation.

The stress from inflammation is another threat to your general health, and PUFAs attack the expression of those genes that encode for factors favorable to inflammation. When your neurons get excited, good things happen. They send signals; process input and allows your brain to function. When they get too excited, though, they are likely to die.

Throughout your life, the brain has to walk a fine line of getting excited and calming down, and they do this using two different neurotransmitter chemicals: GABA (which calms things down) and glutamate (which gets things going). If you tilt more toward excitement, going too far will take you toward such unpleasant destinations as seizures, degenerating neurons and stroke.

The technical term for this is excitotoxicity - the toxic effects of too much excitement. A study from the 1930s found that injecting ketone bodies directly into rabbits kept chemically induced seizures from happening because the ketones kept glutamate from releasing.

However, at the time, the researchers could not identify just why this was the case. More recent studies in neurons of the hippocampus showed that ketones kept neurons from taking on too much glutamate.

Another study showed that the ketogenic diet kept mice from losing cells in the hippocampus by inhibiting the molecules that signal those cells to die. In both rodent and human studies, the ketones boost GABA within the synapses (where neurotransmitters emerge). The result of this is a reduction in the incidence of seizures.

If you're looking for more research involving humans rather than animals, a study involving 23 senior citizens with mild cognitive disorders led to significant improvements in verbal memory after a month and a half on a ketogenic diet.

Another study involved 152 patients who suffered from mild to moderate Alzheimer's disease. For three months, the patients either received an agent with ketones or a placebo while staying with their normal diets. The ones getting the ketogenic drug showed significant improvement in comparison to those receiving the placebo.

A pilot study involving seven Parkinson's disease patients had five who could follow the diet for a month. All of them had a significant reduction in the physical signs of the disease. The most frequent side effects of a ketogenic diet over time appears to include dehydration, constipation and deficiencies in micronutrients and electrolytes.

However, paying attention to hydration often resolves these problems easily. Some patients, usually children, have a higher risk of gallbladder issues, kidney stones and bone fractures.

In women, menstrual irregularities can occur and fertility can suffer as a result. Other than these, no significant side effects have resulted from the ketogenic diet. To be sure, the research shows a need for large scale clinical trials controlled by placebos for patients to see if the ketogenic diet definitely protects the brain.

For people who are using the ketogenic diet for weight loss purposes, having improvements in brain function would certainly be a bonus. However, it is advised to talk to your physician to see if this diet is the right decision for you. No one should make major nutritional changes without talking to one's doctor beforehand. The upside appears to be tremendous, though, in terms of brain health as well as weight loss.

6: Getting Started

Congratulations! You should now have a pretty good understanding of how the ketogenic diet works and now let's get started. The following tips will help you get prepared for success.

Clear out the kitchen

If you tried low carb diet before then you are already familiar with the drill. In a ketogenic diet, carb consumption is ideally around 30-40 grams and almost always below 50. Start by clearing your kitchen of any high carb foods. Again, complex carbohydrates are not allowed so steer clear of them. Put them away for now.

Next, you have to start restocking your kitchen with low carb foods. Stick with vegetables as much as possible. And don't forget about your protein and fat sources too. You don't necessarily have to spend a ton of money on special foods, but when you do your grocery shopping, stick with artificial ingredient-free foods. Choose real foods and forget anything says "low carb". As a rule, if it's marked low carb on the package, you shouldn't be eating it.

In order to keep track of your carb intake, it is recommended that you get yourself a carb counter guide. This will help you monitor your carb consumption with every food or meal you take so you can stay within the limits.

Plan your meals ahead

If you only spend time in the kitchen when eating, you have to change your habit. This diet requires you to spend a little more time in the kitchen. You are encouraged to cook your own meals, which is the best way to keep count of your carb, fat and protein intake.

It is important that you plan your meals ahead of time.

Keep these rules in mind when planning your meals: 60-65 percent of caloric consumption must come from fat, 30 percent should be obtained from protein and the remaining 5-10 percent should consist of carbohydrates.

Drink plenty of water

Since your carb consumption will be reduced, there is a tendency that your kidneys will eliminate excess water it may have held up when you were still eating an unlimited amount of carbs. In which case, it is recommended that you hydrate properly. It is important that you replace the fluids your body lose in the process.

Do not wait until you feel thirsty. Make it a point to drink at least eight glasses of water a day. When you experience muscle cramps and headaches, you are likely losing water. And when you do drink water, you are also advised to take minerals including potassium, magnesium and salt. That's because these minerals get swept away along with water.

Now if you are not too keen about drinking tasteless water, you can always increase your fluid intake through green juices and smoothies. Get juice from high water vegetables such as cucumbers. And you can make smoothies out of any available ingredients around your kitchen. It is also a good way of increasing your vegetable intake.

Don't exercise for the first 2 weeks

This diet puts your body through a lot of changes. You have to give it time to adjust. Do not push yourself to exercise for the first few weeks into the diet. Otherwise, you are only causing unnecessary stress.

What else do you need to know?

As mentioned, you are discouraged from exercising at least for the first few weeks into the diet. The first 2 to 3 weeks are crucial because your body will go through a phase known as the metabolic shift. And during this phase, you should expect to experience brain fog and fatigue.

Watch out for other side effects which may include dizziness, general lethargy and flu-like symptoms. Most of the time, these are signs of dehydration. To increase water retention, you may want to salt everything starting with the water you drink. As your body gets used to the diet and all the changes it brings, these side effects should go away.

Also, because of the limit in carb intake, your body may experience a micronutrient deficiency. This is why you are encouraged to take supplements. Choose a high quality multivitamin with minerals and make sure your body is getting enough fiber by eating plenty of fiber rich green vegetables.

Finally, do not let your blood ketone get out of control. Monitor it regularly. If you go beyond the optimal ketosis level, you are at risk to ketoacidosis.

7: Foods to Eat and Avoid

This dieting program is simple, but you may find it a bit challenging if you are not familiar with it. But then, having a comprehensive knowledge of what foods are suitable or not in the ketogenic diet really makes sense.

Foods to eat

There are food items that take a huge portion of your daily diet. These are the following:

Animal sources (grass-fed)

Lamb, beef, goat and other animal sources of meat is good, but preferably grass-fed. Fish is also an essential, but farmed ones should be avoided. Poultry and pastured pork are also good inclusions in the diet.

Butter, which is basically made from cow's milk, is recommended as it has high omega3 content. Even kidneys, heart and liver of grass-fed animals are perfect for the ketogenic diet.

Fats (healthy)

Always go for saturated ones like clarified butter, coconut oil, lard, poultry fat etc. Oils from nuts and fruits, like avocado is good too as they are monounsaturated along with other polyunsaturated fats or omega 3's coming from fish and other kinds of seafood.

Vegetables

Vegetables are good if you are on a ketogenic diet. However, avoid the starchy ones as they could add up to your carb intake. As much as possible opt for greens like lettuce, spinach and chives as well as cruciferous vegetables like radish. Other good options are; cucumber, celery, eggplant and squash.

Nuts/fruits

Pistachios, macadamia, almonds, cashews, walnuts and other types of nuts are perfect, especially when roasted. But then, you should also keep track of your consumption as anything exceeding the recommended is bad. If you love baking, substitute flax seed flour to the ordinary flour to get fewer carbs.

In terms of beverages, water is always the number one priority. The diet promotes diuresis, so you need to drink at least 8 glasses a day and some more to prevent dehydration. Apart from water, you may also consume tea and coffee, but avoid sodas and anything that is loaded with artificial sweeteners.

Foods to avoid

In the ketogenic diet, there are just some foods that you should totally avoid. Take a look below to get the best idea:

Grains

All types of grains like corn, rice, wheat, barley, soy, quinoa and other food items produced by grains such as pasta, bread, crackers should be avoided. Sweets and sugary foods like cakes, ice creams and pastries must be removed from the diet too.

Farmed animals

Surely, pork, beef and chicken are allowed on the ketogenic diet. However, you should avoid farmed fish as they are high in fatty acids omega 6 which can inflame the body. Farmed fish may contain substances like mercury that is bad for your body.

Anything processed

Processed foods like almond milk, gelatin, dried fruits as well as instant meals are not good if you are trying to lose weight on the ketogenic diet. Also, those that are labeled "0 carbs", "low-fat" or "low carbs", such as in diet soft drinks, mints and gums must be avoided.

Fruits

Fruits are allowed in the diet, but you should stay away from tropical ones, such as pineapple, papaya, mangoes and plantains since they have high carb content. Say "no" to fruit juices as well as they are rich in sugar. Instead, go for fruit smoothies as they are rich in fiber and more filling.

Milk

Though milk is also a source of protein, it should be consumed moderately, especially high fat and raw ones. Milk is hard to digest and it has high carb content: 100ml of high-fat milk contains about 5 grams of carbs. If you love milk with your tea or coffee, settle for cream instead.

Sweet beverage and alcohol

Artificial sweeteners in various commercially available beverages are not ketogenic diet friendly as well as alcoholic drinks. Remember, you are trying to avoid as much sugar as possible in this diet, so why load your body with this stuff?

A few more words on fruits and vegetables

Many people think that simply adding a regimen of fruits and vegetables to their diet will make the pounds melt off. It's true that pineapple is a more nutritious snack than potato chips, but pineapple has a lot of calories too, in the form of fructose (the sugar that is found in fruits).

There are even some vegetables that are fairly high in carbs, which can be a trap for people trying to lose weight with a low carb diet. This section contains a list of some of the more common low carb fruits and vegetables, in rough order from lowest to highest in terms of carbs per serving.

However, all of the foods on this list are low in carbs and will work well on a ketogenic diet.

Alfalfa sprouts

Throwing these on top of a salad gives you a bit more fiber without adding much at all in the way of starches or carbs. However, legumes with sprouts tend to have a little more in the way of carbs.

Greens

Fill your plate with spinach, chard, lettuce and other similar greens. You might have to add some other foods to provide enough flavor to make this a palatable option, but greens are basically roughage that also help you get some key nutrients, such as iron. You can eat as much of these as you want, because the caloric and carb input is minimal.

Hearty greens

These are things like kale, mustard greens and collard greens. There is a little more flavor with these dishes, but you also get some more carbs in the mix even though you are still fine on the ketogenic index.

Herbs

You don't have to just garnish it on your plate, as basil, cilantro, thyme, rosemary and other herbs add a good bit of flavor to your meals. If having some more spinach just doesn't sound appetizing, try throwing some of these herbs on top of your food. It can make your meal look a lot more attractive.

Bok Choy

Also known as Pak Choi, or Chinese cabbage, this vegetable belongs in the brassica family with the other cabbages. There are fewer carbs in this variety than there are in the typical round cabbages you see in the grocery store.

Look for the dark leaves and the long white stalks. When it is in season, there is a smaller variety called bok choy that is a bit more tender. Either way, this is a nutritious vegetable with minimal carbs.

Celery

This is a low carb vegetable that is quite versatile, usable in soups as well as a stand-alone snack, with cream cheese or peanut butter as an accompaniment. With some more flavor than some of the other vegetables on this list, celery is one of the more popular low carb vegetables.

Brussels sprouts

These are an acquired taste that often requires significant seasoning and butter to make it palatable. The good news is that butter and seasonings are two things that people on the ketogenic diet can have, so be creative with the way you prepare these veggies.

Snow peas

These are cool and crunchy when are served raw while retaining their crispy texture when you add them to a stir fry. The pleasant flavor makes this a favorite among ketogenic eaters.

Tomatoes

These red vegetables are bursting with flavor as well as the nutrient lycopene. Low in carbs, tomatoes are an excellent source of snack. After slicing it into small wedges, you can sprinkle them on crackers for a nutritious snack.

You're going to have fewer choices when it comes to fruits than you will with vegetables because all fruits contain fructose, a sugar that contributes to their sweet flavor. However, there are a number of fruits that you can incorporate into your diet. These appear roughly in order from lowest to highest in terms of carbohydrates.

Lemon/Lime

Obviously, you won't be cutting these up and eating them, but adding portions to drinks gives you some added flavor without adding much of anything to your carb count. If you're trying to drink more water, then adding a slice of one of these can make it a lot more palatable.

Raspberries

High in antioxidants, raspberries are a fairly tart fruit that nonetheless adds freshness to your plate. Blackberries and cranberries are actually good choices as well. All of these have a ton of fiber, minerals and vitamins, in addition to those antioxidants that promote better health, and may even keep you from developing heart disease and cancer as time goes by. There are some researchers that believe that these antioxidants even slow down the process of aging. It just takes a cup to give you your entire day's required portion of Vitamin C.

Strawberries

These have a little more sugar than the other berries, but unless you add whipped cream or syrup, you're not taking in too many carbs to make these a solid idea on the ketogenic diet.

Watermelon

Particularly popular in the summertime, watermelons are a great way to keep yourself hydrated while also getting the dietary fiber that fruit provides. You can't eat as much of these as you can the berries, because of the sugar involved, but you can add smaller portions to your plate.

Peaches and nectarines

These are about as high as you want to go in terms of sugars when you're on the ketogenic diet. Also in season during the summer, these are a great way to satisfy your sweet tooth without undoing the good of your ketogenic eating plan.

Shopping tips

Some people say that the ketogenic diet is an expensive choice, but this is not the case. In fact, you can enjoy the goodness and the benefits of this diet without having to spend a fortune.

Follow these tips:

Take advantage of coupons

Couponing is such a fad these days, and this is because these little pieces of paper that you see online or in the newspaper pages can help you get tremendous savings on your purchase.

Buy food in bulk

Since you have an idea of the types of food that you should eat, it is best to buy them in bulk and simply place them in your freezer to prolong its shelf life. Doing this will also give you less stress since you've got everything that you need right in the fridge.

Make your own food

Surely, the peanut butter and garlic ranch salad dressing that you can get straight from the shelf of grocery stores are yummy. However, you can make this stuff in your kitchen. If you do, you can benefit from extra delicious and healthier food products in just a fraction of a price compared to the ones that are ready-made.

Go to farmer's market once in a while

Food products like meats and natural produce are cheaper when purchased in the farmer's market. Plus, these items are organic too! You will not only save money but you will be able to stay away from toxins present in non-organic food products.

8: A Sample Diet Plan

Overall, the ketogenic diet can be described as eating meat in controlled portions, low carb foods, and high-fat foods. But deciding what to eat each day can be difficult especially if you are a beginner.

Day 1

Breakfast

Powdered whey protein mixed with 400ml almond milk (unsweetened) and 4 tablespoons of heavy cream.

Lunch

3 to 4 ounces smoked meat

1 cup of squash cooked in olive oil

1 handful of lettuce with vinegar or olive oil dressing

Unsweetened beverage/water

Dinner

3 to 4 ounces baked pink salmon with cream sauce

1 1/2 cups of spinach cooked in oil, garlic and onions

1 cup of lettuce with high fat salad dressing

Water/coffee with cream or any unsweetened beverage

Day 2

Breakfast

3 eggs scrambled with chives

Slice of pastured ham cooked in a tablespoon of lard

2 cups spinach with mushroom and cherry tomatoes

Water/coffee topped with cream/tea

Lunch

4 to 5 ounces stewed pork

2 cups of chard in high-fat dressing or 2 tablespoons of homemade dressing

A pinch of Himalayan salt

Water/unsweetened beverage

Dinner

250 g pan fried in a spoon of ghee and a pinch of salt

1 cup of iceberg lettuce with lemon juice or vinegar dressing

Water, tea/coffee

Day 3

Breakfast

1/2 cup of berries (strawberry, blackberries)

a handful of nuts (macadamia or almonds)

3/4 cup coconut milk

Water

Combine everything the night before and put in the fridge.

Lunch

1 to 2 cups of iceberg lettuce with 3/4 cup canned tuna, 2 boiled eggs, 2 tablespoons of home-made mayonnaise and a dash of salt or citrus

Unsweetened beverage/smoothie

Dinner

3 to 4 ounces crispy bacon

1 cup spinach with garlic mayo dressing

2 eggs fried in lard or ghee

Creamed coffee, water or tea

Day 4

Breakfast

2 eggs fried in ghee

1 big slice of ham

1 cup blanched spinach

1/2 avocado fruit

Water/coffee or tea

Lunch

1/2 cup of boiled chicken

2 cups romaine lettuce or chard

1 whole avocado sliced thinly

2 tablespoon mayo-mustard dressing

Water/unsweetened sparkling drink

Dinner

1 medium sized lamb chops seasoned with a pinch of salt, pan fried in ghee

1 cup of green beans sautéed in olive oil or butter

Water/ spiced tea

Day 5

Breakfast

Whey protein smoothie with 3 to 4 tablespoon heavy cream

1/2 cup berries

Lunch

4 ounces chicken breast pan friend in a tablespoon of butter

2 cups romaine lettuce with 2 tablespoon ranch dressing

Unsweetened beverage/water

Dinner

4 ounces rib eye beef steak pan friend in 2 tablespoons salted butter

1 cup raw broccoli with 2 tablespoons of heavy sour cream as a dip

Spiced tea/water/unsweetened sparkling

Day 6

Breakfast

1 egg boiled or fried

4 ounces pastured ham

1/2 cup braised spinach

1/2 cup blackberries/raspberry

Water/tea

Lunch

250g prawns roasted in 1 tablespoon of ghee, a pinch of cayenne pepper and salt

1 1/2 cup of chard with 2 tablespoons of oil dressing (olive oil)

Water/tea

Dinner

1 medium sized pork chop pan fried in 1-2 tablespoons salted butter

1 cup lettuce with 4 ounces cherry tomatoes, 1 ounce spring onion with olive oil and salt

Creamed coffee, lemon juice or water

Day 7

Breakfast

3 eggs cooked omelet style and topped with ground meat

150 grams sauerkraut

Water/coffee with cream/tea

Lunch

1/2 cup thinly sliced avocado with a cup of lettuce, 2 hard-boiled eggs, salt and olive oil

Dinner

4 ounces pan roasted salmon in a tablespoon of ghee or lard in hollandaise sauce

1 bunch of pan-fried asparagus

Water/unsweetened sparkling beverage

Snacks

For snacks, you may opt for celery sticks, kimchi, hard-boiled eggs, ham rolls, nuts and seeds, berries, bone broth and pork cracklings among others.

All the sample menus presented above ranges from 1500 to 2000 kilocalories a day and follow the ideal distribution of macronutrients in a ketogenic diet: 60% fat, 30% protein and 10% carbs.

Do's and don'ts

To make the ketogenic work for you, it is best that you know the common mistakes to avoid and the best practices that must be observed. Remember, this program will only work if done correctly.

Do's

Watch out for carbs

Take this thing seriously since eating too many carbs will only ruin your goal. Beware of carb rich and starchy foods as well as processed items. Well, this may be hard especially if you love to eat rice, pasta, potatoes and bread. However, there are still your eggs, bacon, lamb, beef, heavy creams and nuts.

So, why not be happy with berries and non-starchy veggies as your sources of carbs? This should make sense if you really want to start burning body fats.

Eat protein in moderation

Though you have much freedom to consume protein in a low carb diet, make sure that you do not over-do it. If you eat too much, the excess protein will be converted to glucose, which may hinder your body from getting into the state of ketosis.

Consume fat

Don't be scared of eating fat since you need the fat to fuel your body since you already removed most of the carbs in your diet. This should constitute around 60% of your total caloric intake.

To do this, make sure you eat fatty meat cuts and a generous amount of healthy fats such as coconut oil, butter, olive oil, ghee and lard to your diet.

Don'ts

Don't forget to replenish salt

You will be losing a lot of sodium when you are on the ketogenic diet. Therefore, you should recharge with sodium or else you will suffer from headaches, dizziness, fatigue and digestive problems. So be liberal with adding salt to your food and drink one cup of broth a day if you feel your body needs it.

Don't stay away from fruits and vegetables

Many people think that fruits and vegetables should be removed during the ketogenic diet. It is true that some fruits and veggies are starchy or sugary, but there are those that are rich in fiber and nutrients that will help the body fight inflammation and make you feel satiated after each meal. The secret is to know which fruits and vegetables are allowed and which are prohibited.

Don't rush

Always be patient. Generally, it takes 3 to 5 days for your body to achieve the state of ketosis. So, stick to the low carb diet as much as possible, especially in the beginning to allow your body to get into the metabolic adaptation. However, you should take it gradually. Do not cut down on your carb intake abruptly as this could confuse your body and may cause harm.

9: Ketogenic Recipes

Breakfast

Breakfast is the most important meal of the day and this principle also applies with the ketogenic diet. Whether you are in a hurry or have a little time to spare for breakfast, you will absolutely enjoy the following recipes. You will surely find one that matches the kind of morning you are having.

Sausage patties

Free from gluten and soy content, this breakfast sausage is perfectly fit for someone trying to lose weight. It is easy and you can make it ahead of time *and* store in the refrigerator. This recipe yields 15 servings.

Ingredients:

- 2 pounds of ground chicken sausage
- 1/4 cup of white finely chopped onion
- 3 garlic cloves, finely minced
- 1 tablespoon of ground sage
- 1/2 tablespoon of finely minced rosemary
- 1 tablespoon salt
- 1/2 tablespoon freshly ground black pepper

Put all the ingredients in a large bowl. Mix well until the seasonings are well combined with the meat. Divide the mixture into 7 equal portions. You can use an ice cream scoop for this process. Press on the mixture to form a patty.

Arrange the patties on a waxed cookie sheet. Store the patties by stacking them together, separating one from the other by placing a paper after each patty layer. Then, cover the entire stack using a plastic wrap. Place in the fridge for at least 2 hours.

You can cook these sausage patties immediately after taking them out of the fridge. Use a lidded pan for cooking over medium heat. Each side of the patty must be cooked for 6 or 7 minutes.

Breakfast casserole

The usual casserole recipes are filled with cheese, making them fattening. This casserole recipe is not only a much healthier alternative, it is also very delicious. The only downside is it takes some time to prepare and cook. You need to spare a total of 55 minutes for both prep and cooking. This recipe yields 2 servings.

Ingredients:

- 5 eggs
- 3 bacon strips, cooked
- 1 cup fresh baby spinach
- 1/2 cup butternut squash, chopped

- 1/2 cup fresh mushrooms, sliced
- 1/2 cup yellow squash, chopped
- 1/4 cup red onion, chopped
- 1 pinch garlic powder
- Salt and pepper to taste

Pre-heat the oven first to 350 degrees. Combine all the ingredients in a medium sized bowl except for the seasoning. Mix well. Next, add garlic powder with salt and pepper to taste.

Brush the bottom and sides of the baking dish with coconut oil. Pour the mixture. Put inside the pre-heated oven. Let it cook at 350 degrees for 45 minutes. When cooked, place in a cooling rack, and then serve.

Chia breakfast

This breakfast recipe is ideal for busy mornings. If you're used to oatmeal, this is your healthier option. It's so easy to prepare, it will only take ten minutes or less of your time. This recipe is good for two.

Ingredients:

- 1 cup boiling water
- 1/2 cup almond milk, unsweetened
- 4 tablespoons of Chia seeds
- 4 tablespoons shredded coconut, unsweetened
- 4 tablespoons flax meal

- 1 tablespoon cinnamon
- Stevia

Mix all the ingredients in a bowl except for the water and almond milk. Make sure the mixture is well blended. Now pour the boiling water into the mixture. Stir it well. Set it aside for 3 minutes then stir.

Add the almond milk then stir and serve.

Spinach and mushroom quiche

This is another easy breakfast recipe you can make in 40 minutes. This recipe serves two.

Ingredients:

- 6 large eggs
- 3 white mushrooms, sliced
- 1/2 medium onion, finely chopped
- 1 cup of chopped fresh spinach
- 1/2 cup unsweetened almond milk
- 1/2 teaspoon baking powder
- Salt and pepper

Preheat the oven to 350 degrees Fahrenheit. Beat the eggs in a bowl then add the coconut milk. Whisk together using a hand mixer. Add the rest of the ingredients one by one as you continue stirring.

Apply grease on a baking dish. Pour the quiche mixture into the baking dish then bake for about 40 minutes. You can take this breakfast dish to go by slicing the quiche into squares before storing them in a Ziploc bag.

Low carb breakfast bar

This is one of the most convenient breakfast recipes in the list. You can make this breakfast in less than 20 minutes. This recipe yields 5 servings.

Ingredients:

- 1 large egg
- 1/4 creamy roasted almond butter
- 1/2 tablespoon cinnamon
- 1/2 teaspoon vanilla
- 1/4 teaspoon baking soda
- Sea salt
- Stevia

Put the almond butter in a medium sized bowl and blend until creamy. Add egg, vanilla, honey and stevia then stir. You can also use a blender to make sure the ingredients are well blended. Then, add grease to a baking dish. Pour the batter into the dish and put in the oven. Let it cook at 325 degrees Fahrenheit for 12 to 15 minutes. Place in a cooling rack then divide into 5 equal portions. Enjoy!

Coconut pudding with chia

Chia is a reliable ingredient for low carb recipes on the go. The gelatinous texture of the chia combined with the softness of blueberry is a match made in heaven. Add a little Stevia to sweeten. The natural sweetness of the berries with the flavoring of vanilla is enough to make this a breakfast delight. This recipe is good for one.

For the ingredients, you need the following:

- 2 tablespoons chia seed
- 2 tablespoons unsweet coconut
- 1/2 cup water
- 1/2 teaspoon vanilla

Put the chia seeds, coconut, water and vanilla in the blender. Process the ingredients until smooth. Pour the mixture into a bowl. Let it cool in the fridge for 15 to 30 minutes or until you have a thick mixture. Take it out.

For additional flavor, you can also sprinkle the pudding with nuts.

Cucumber and strawberry salad

This breakfast is perfect for a lazy Sunday morning. It is especially good when the weather is hot. This refreshing salad is ideal as a light breakfast or side dish to a grilled food. This recipe serves two.

Ingredients:

- 1/2 cucumber, peeled and sliced
- 2 fresh strawberries, sliced
- 1/2 green bell pepper, diced
- 2 tablespoons freshly squeezed lime juice
- Sesame seeds

Put the green bell pepper in a small bowl and drizzle with lime juice. Mix well. Combine the strawberries and cucumber in the bowl and mix. Then, add the pepper and lime mixture.

Toss until ingredients are well coated. Let it chill in the fridge for a few minutes. Sprinkle with sesame seeds before serving. If you like your breakfast with a creamy flavor, feel free to add feta cheese.

Lunch

You need time to plan your lunch ahead. When you prepare in advance, you can choose healthier options as well as save money. Make sure you have healthy ingredients on hand.

Make sure your lunch is packed with protein to help fill you up. Protein also makes you feel satisfied for a longer period of time. Choose lean protein sources. Use a variety of fruits and vegetables as ingredients too. That said, below is a list of lunch recipes that are both nutritious and delicious.

Bulgarian ground meat

This recipe adds a whole new meaning to dieting. The mix of herbs and spices lends an interesting flavor to the meat. Add a fresh side salad to this and it is one you will love.

Ingredients:

- 1/4 pound ground beef
- 1 egg
- 1/2 onion, chopped
- 1/4 tablespoon dried thyme
- Ginger, coriander and ground cumin
- Salt and pepper to taste

Combine the ingredients in a large bowl. If you feel the mixture requires additional eggs, feel free to add. Scoop the mixture into the bread slices. Put it in the oven and bake the sandwich at medium heat for 7 minutes or until the meat is cooked through. Serve and enjoy!

Crab cakes

The key to successful dieting is variety. Here's a sumptuous crab cake recipe you will surely enjoy.

Ingredients:

- 1/2 pound crab meat
- 1 medium egg
- 1/8 cup breadcrumbs (made from almond flour)
- 1 tablespoon olive oil
- 1 tablespoon mayonnaise
- 1/2 tablespoon diced celery
- 1/2 tablespoon minced onion
- 1/4 tablespoon minced garlic
- 1/2 teaspoon Old Bay Seasoning
- 1/2 teaspoon Dijon mustard
- Salt and pepper

Combine the ingredients in a large bowl without the breadcrumbs and crab meat. Mix well then add crab meat. Mix again then gradually add the breadcrumbs.

Scoop the mixture into equal portions. Shape each portion into a ball and flatten to form cakes with half inch thickness.

Heat the pan and add olive oil. When the oil is hot enough, cook the crab cakes until each side is golden brown. Cook two cakes at a time. Serve immediately!

Thai style shrimp salad

If you are craving a little spice, you will absolutely love this Thai recipe. A well balanced flavor with just the right amount of spice, this salad is surely satisfying. This recipe is good for two.

Ingredients:

- 1/2 pound steamed shrimp, cleaned and deveined
- 1/2 head lettuce, cut into small pieces
- 1/2 stalk lemongrass, sliced
- 1 red onion, sliced
- 1/4 inch ginger root, cut into small pieces
- 1 fresh red chili, sliced
- 1 garlic clove, crushed and minced
- 7 mint leaves
- 1 and 1/2 teaspoon lime juice
- 2 tablespoons chopped green onions
- 2 tablespoons chopped fresh cilantro
- 1 tablespoon fish sauce
- Black pepper

Lay the lettuce leaves flat and arrange the shrimp over it. Pour the ginger, chili and onion on top. Set aside.

In the meantime, prepare the dressing. Combine the lime juice, lemongrass, garlic, pepper, and fish sauce together in a bowl. Mix well then pour over the shrimp salad. Add the cilantro, onion and mint leaves to garnish and serve.

Mexican ceviche

This seafood dish is commonly served on the beaches of Mexico. It is best served with sweet potato, lettuce or avocado and other side dishes that can complement its interesting flavors. If you want something different from your usual lunch, you have to give this dish a shot. And when you do, make sure you only use the freshest ingredients. This recipe is good for one.

Ingredients:

- 1/4 pound halibut fillet
- 1 lime
- 1 jalapeno pepper, finely chopped
- 1/2 small onion, finely chopped
- 1/4 green bell pepper, finely chopped
- 1/4 cup fresh tomato, finely sliced
- 1 tablespoon chopped parsley
- 1/2 chopped fresh cilantro
- 1/2 tablespoon white vinegar
- 1/8 teaspoon oregano
- Salt and pepper
- Lettuce leaf
- Avocado and black olives for garnishing

Cut the fish into pieces. Each piece should be about half an inch. Squeeze lime juice over the fish. Stir. Then, store in the fridge overnight.

Before lunchtime, take the fish out and drain. Add the rest of the ingredients except for the avocado, lettuce and olives. Toss well. Arrange the lettuce on a serving dish. Lay it flat and pour the fish mixture over it. Add the black olives and avocado slices for garnishing. Serve and enjoy!

Black bean garlic sauce with Brussels sprouts

The flavor of the black bean garlic sauce goes perfectly well with the sprouts. There is no need to add salt because the sauce itself adds just enough flavor. If you want to try a little taste of Asian food, this recipe is a good way to start. You can easily find the sauce in your local grocery's Asian aisle. This recipe serves one.

Ingredients:

- 1/4 pound Brussels sprouts
- 1/2 tablespoon black bean garlic sauce
- 1/2 tablespoon extra virgin olive oil
- Black pepper

Before you start, make sure the Brussels sprouts are cleaned well. Next, trim and cut them lengthwise.

Place a skillet over medium high heat and pour oil. Add the sprouts and toss. Let it cook for 3 minutes or until they turn brown.

Next, pour the black bean garlic sauce over the sprouts. Stir until evenly coated. Add black pepper and cook for about 30 seconds more. Serve immediately.

Sesame salmon salad

Packed with salmon flavor with the goodness of sesame, you will surely love this recipe. You can enjoy this salad either warm or cold, it is just as good. It can be served as a light main meal or as lunch. This recipe makes 2 servings.

Ingredients:

- 1/2 pound wild sockeye salmon fillet
- 4 won ton wrappers
- 2 green onions, finely chopped
- 1 egg
- 1 small avocado, cut lengthwise
- 1/2 small head napa cabbage, cut into pieces
- 1/8 pound trimmed and blanched snow peas
- 1/2 tablespoon sesame seeds
- 1/8 cup cilantro, chopped
- Vegetable oil
- Lemongrass

- Chile dressing
- Salt

Cut the salmon into half-an-inch thick pieces, and then put in a pot of simmering water with salt. Cover and cook for 5 minutes. Once cooked, drain, take the gray layer underneath it out and set aside to cool.

Put the vegetables into a large pot. Pour oil and place over a medium heat. Set aside once cooked.

Crack the egg into a bowl and add 1 tablespoon of water. Whisk well. Use the egg wash for brushing each side the won tons. Sprinkle with sesame seeds and fry until golden and puffy. Place the cooked won ton on a paper towel then sprinkle with salt.

Place the orange slices, snow peas, cilantro, green onions and cabbage in a large bowl. Pour the dressing and toss. Transfer into serving dishes and place cooked salmon on the side with the avocado slices and fried won ton dishes. Add cilantro leaves to garnish.

Dinner

Your dinner recipes should also provide you with enough protein and a sufficient amount of nutrients. The following is a list of healthy recipes that can help keep you energized and feeling full to avoid hunger pangs and emotional cravings. If you are longing for a light and comforting dinner, you can have a sumptuous soup too.

Chicken and mushrooms

Chicken and mushrooms do not just make a great pair in a creamy soup. They are also a perfect match when it comes to a main dish.

This recipe is good for one. Ingredients:

- 1 boneless chicken breast
- 1 cup sliced mushrooms
- 1/4 cup chopped green bell pepper
- 1 1/2 tablespoon soy sauce
- 1/4 tablespoon minced onion
- 1/2 teaspoon honey
- Garlic powder

Preheat the oven to 350 degrees Fahrenheit. Place the boneless chicken breast on a baking dish. Top with onion flakes.

Mix the soy sauce with the garlic powder in a bowl and pour over the chicken. Cover the baking dish. Place in the pre-heated oven. Let the chicken cook for 30 minutes.

Once cooked, uncover the baking dish and add mushrooms and bell pepper on top. Cover the dish again and place it back inside the oven. Bake until the mushrooms are tender. Take it out and set aside to cool. Serve.

Low carb turkey meatballs

This recipe has an Italian ring to it. Not your usual meatball recipe that uses beef or pork. Rather, this dish's main attraction is turkey! It is only at 166 calories and it is not even that hard to make. This recipe makes 3 meatballs.

Ingredients:

- 1/2 pound ground turkey
- 1 egg
- 1 garlic clove, finely minced
- 1/8 cup breadcrumbs (made from almond flour)
- 1/8 cup of chopped onion
- 1/8 cup chopped parsley
- 1/4 teaspoon oregano
- Salt and pepper

Mix all the ingredients in a large bowl. Divide into three equal portions. Shape each portion into round balls then flatten. Place a non-stick pan over medium heat and spray with oil. Cook each side of the meatballs for about 6 minutes or until brown and cooked through. Serve immediately.

Cajun halibut

This is a simple way of cooking halibut steaks. The Cajun flavor mixes well with the fish. It is a sumptuous treat for dinner. This recipe serves two.

Ingredients:

- 2 halibut steaks
- 1/8 teaspoon each of ground red pepper, ground black pepper, garlic powder, paprika and salt

Combine the seasonings in a small bowl. Rub both sides of halibut with the seasoning mixture.

Place non-stick skillet over a medium heat. Apply cooking spray then add fish. Cook each side of the halibut for 4 minutes or until cooked through. Serve immediately.

Baked chicken thighs

This is one juicy chicken recipe. And the best part is that it does not call for a heavy prep. This recipe is best served with mixed vegetables and rice, and garnished with chopped fresh parsley. This recipe is good for two.

Ingredients:

- 2 chicken thighs

- 2 tablespoons soy sauce
- Garlic powder

Arrange the chicken on a baking dish then sprinkle with garlic powder and pour with soy sauce. Place in the oven and cook at 350 degrees Fahrenheit for about an hour.

Beef with broccoli

This stir fry recipe is Chinese inspired. If you want an unusually tasty and delicious dish using simple and easy to find ingredients, this is your best bet. You can enjoy this stir fry with hot brown rice. This recipe is good for one.

Ingredients:

1/4 pound round steak, cut into thick strips

1/4 onion, sliced into wedges

1 cup broccoli florets

1/8 cup water

1 tablespoon cornstarch

1 tablespoon of soy sauce

1 tablespoon vegetable oil

1 tablespoon water, divided

1/4 teaspoon ground ginger

1/8 teaspoon garlic powder

Mix garlic powder with half a tablespoon each of cornstarch and water together in a bowl and add the beef strips. Mix well.

Place a skillet over medium heat and pour half the oil portion. Add coated beef strips and stir fry until tender. Transfer the beef strips on a plate. Then, pour other half portion of oil into the skillet and cook the onion and broccoli. Cook for 4 minutes. Add the beef strips back into the skillet and pour brown sugar, ginger, cornstarch, soy sauce and water. Stir fry for another 2 minutes. Serve immediately.

Sautéed shrimp

This is one tasty dish. It goes well with roasted vegetables. This shrimp recipe serves two.

Ingredients:

- 1/2 pound shrimp, peeled and deveined
- 1 tablespoon freshly squeezed lemon juice
- 1 tablespoon chopped parsley
- 1 teaspoon of olive oil
- 1/2 teaspoon herb seasoning
- Salt and pepper

Place skillet over a medium heat and pour oil. Stir in shrimp and sauté for 1 minute. Sprinkle with salt, herb seasoning and pepper. Drizzle with lemon juice and keep stirring. Cook for 4 minutes more. Sprinkle chopped parsley before transferring to a serving dish.

Lemony chicken soup

A yummy soup that can provide comfort especially in cold weather, this is a perfect way to end a long week. You can make it so the soup forms drops by not stirring the eggs. But if you want something different from an egg drop soup, stir in the egg so it does not form. This recipe makes 3 to 4 servings.

Ingredients:

- 1 cup of cooked chicken, cut into half inch thick pieces
- 1 cup chicken broth
- 1 egg
- 1 chicken bouillon cube
- 1 sliced carrot
- 1/2 small onion, minced
- 1 tablespoon freshly squeezed lemon juice
- Oregano
- Salt and pepper

Place the chicken broth, chicken bouillon cube and 1 cup water into a Dutch oven. Let it boil the chicken. Simmer for 20 minutes. Pour in lemon juice along with the egg. Sprinkle with salt, pepper and oregano. Serve while hot.

10: FAQ

How can people get into ketosis?

The quickest way to reach ketosis is through limiting carbohydrates within range of 20 to 50 grams each day or lesser than 10% of your total calories for the day. Some low-carb dieters take very small portions of carbohydrates, usually not reaching five percent of their total daily calories intake.

Also, specific exercise techniques and diet, like HUT or High Intensity Interval Training and intermittent abstaining from food assist getting into ketosis quickly and make losing fat efficient and easy.

What are the advantages of ketosis?

The obvious advantage of ketosis is improved lipid loss. What healthier way of sculpting that flab from your physique than burning it away as power? To ensure this, have fewer calories as compared to your energy needs. There are also medical motives for engaging in and continuing in ketosis, such as for management of epilepsy and as an alternative cancer therapy.

What are the disadvantages of ketosis?

The main problem with ketosis remains that certain people refuse to believe that top athletes could get adequate energy from being in ketosis. These happen to be people having high-energy occupations that do similar exercises, people who toil at work a great deal or high-level players.

Another downfall with ketosis is extremely restrictive manner to dine and countless people have issues adhering towards the proper nourishment. Also, a lasting, low-carb intake may injure the metabolic rate, particularly one combined with a little calorie supply and extreme cardio workout. Some individuals may proceed with the low carbohydrate sequence too long, removing all vegetables and fruits in the process.

Fruits and vegetables provide minerals and vitamins essential towards good fitness, and possess anti-oxidants. Thus, if you attempt ketosis to burn fat, ensure you perform your study and try not to cut down too much on fruits and veggies.

How could you drop weight through eating fat?

Ketogenic meal plans of 50 grams of carbohydrates a day remain extremely operational for becoming lean. By consuming fat, you rearrange the enzymatic gear to utilize fat and to make it become a way of its prime fuel.

There are, however, three issues with your food and drink which may affect your fat loss; excessive protein, inadequate good fats, and leftover carbohydrates.

How much carbs should a person eat? How much is "low"?

We are all different and whatever is extreme for you might not be the same for somebody else. The best way to find out is to check how you feel. If you find yourself tired and sleepy after eating, you probably had too much carbohydrates and, therefore, you experience a sudden increase of insulin level.

The problem is, by elevating your sugar in your blood, you become hungrier. This will make you eat more than usual. Unless the extra carbohydrates you take are part of the ketosis diet meal plan, you must avoid taking too much carbs. Certain people cannot eat in excess of 10 grams of net carbohydrates per mealtime while other people do not experience significant spikes in their insulin at much higher level like 50 grams of net carbohydrates.

How long does it take for an average healthy person to enter the ketosis state?

It takes about 72 hours with the effort of low-carb pattern of eating. Lean meat, colorful vegetables, healthful carbs, such as sweet potato and brown rice, is a far healthier and far more nutritious.

Moreover, depriving yourself of tasty food is simply not amusing and, like the remaining portion of your life, balance is the key towards success.

Is ketosis safe? What are the possible dangers of ketosis, if any?

Ketosis is safe, but aligned with other circumstances, well, it varies.

If anyone tells you that being in ketosis is dangerous for you, they are most likely confusing nutritional ketosis with diabetic ketoacidosis (DKA is a medical term that's used to describe a life-threatening condition in type 1 diabetics).

Many doctors will discourage their patients from getting into a state of ketosis because they immediately think of all the negative side effects associated with ketoacidosis, but they are ignorant of all the benefits.

Ketoacidosis can cause type 1 diabetics to become very dehydrated, which causes the blood to become acidic and ketone levels to shoot up to levels of 25 or higher. With nutritional ketosis, such as this diet promotes, ketone levels are usually much lower and safer.

What foods can be freely be eaten under the ketogenic diet?

Consume freely grass-fed and wild animal resources:

- Ghee, grass-fed venison, lamb, beef, goat, wild-caught seafood and fish, pastured poultry, eggs and pork; gelatin and butter, since they are rich in beneficial omega 3 fatty acids.
- Avoid hot dogs, sausages, farmed fish, meat covered with breadcrumbs and that goes with sweet or starch sauces;
- Grass-fed offal like heart, liver, kidneys and other meat of animal organ.

Wholesome lipids:

- Saturated fat: butter, tallow, lard, chicken, duck and goose fat, clarified butter or ghee, and coconut oil;

- Monounsaturated fat: olive oil, macadamia, avocado;
- Polyunsaturated omega 3, expressly from animal origins like fatty seafood and fish;
- Avoid high-heat preparing for these foods.

Non-starchy vegetables:

- Green leafy vegetables, for example: chives, lettuce, Bok choy, Swiss chard, spinach, chard, endive or radicchio;
- Some cruciferous veggies, like dark leaf kale, kohlrabi or radishes;
- Spaghetti squash, asparagus, celery stalk, cucumber, zucchini, or bamboo shoots.

Fruits, nuts and seeds:

- Coconut, avocado and macadamia nuts.

Drinks and condiments:

- Water, black coffee or coffee with cream or coconut milk, and black or herbal tea;
- Cracklings for food coating;
- Home-produced bone broth, mustard, mayonnaise, pesto, pickles, kimchi, and sauerkraut, as homemade products have no preservatives or coloring;
- All herbs and spices, and lime or lemon zest and juice;

- Whey and egg white protein, and hormone-free, grass-fed gelatin;
- Be careful of soy lecithin, additives, non-natural sweeteners and hormones.

What foods can be occasionally eaten under the ketogenic diet?

Vegetables, mushrooms and fruits:

- Some cruciferous veggies, such as turnips, Brussels sprouts, broccoli, green, red and white cabbage, cauliflower, fennel, rutabaga or swede;
- Nightshades, like tomatoes, eggplant and peppers;
- Some root veggies, for example, mushrooms, onions, spring onion, parsley root, leek, garlic, winter squash or pumpkin;
- Sea vegetables, such as wax beans, sugar snap peas, bean sprouts, nori, kombu, okra, French or globe artichokes, and water chestnuts;
- Rhubarb, olives and berries, like mulberries, raspberries, blueberries, blackberries, strawberries and cranberries.

Dairy and grain-fed animal resources:

- Poultry, ghee, beef and eggs;
- Avoid farmed pig meat as it is too rich in omega 6;

- Dairy products, such as sour cream, cottage cheese, plain full-fat yogurt, cream and cheese;
- Avoid products tagged as low-fat as mostly are filled with starch and sugar, besides having little satisfying effect;
- Bacon, except those with preservatives, as well as added starch.

Seeds and nuts:

- Pumpkin and sesame seeds, pine nuts, walnuts, pecans, almonds, hazelnuts, flax seed, sunflower and hemp seeds;
- Brazil nuts, except those having very elevated selenium level.

Fermented products from soy:

- Eat only non-GMO and fermented products from soy, such as soy sauce, Tempeh, Natto or paleo-friendly coconut aminos.
- Unprocessed black soybeans and Edamame or green soy beans.

Condiments:

- Healthy carb-free sweeteners, such as Stevia, Erythritol or Swerve;
- Thickeners: powdered arrowroot or xanthan gum;

- Sugar-free products from tomato, like puree, passata or ketchup;
- Cocoa and powdered carob, cocoa powder, or extra dark chocolate;
- Beware of mints, soy lecithin and sugar-free masticating gums as some have carbohydrates.

Some vegetables, fruits, nuts and seeds with average carbohydrates:

- Root vegetables, such as sweet potato, parsnip, carrot, celery root and beetroot;
- Fresh cherries, oranges, grapefruit, nectarine, apricot, watermelon, cantaloupe, Gallia, honeydew melons, Pitaya or dragon fruit, peach, apple, kiwi fruit and berries, plums, pears and figs;
- Dried fruit, like berries, dates, raisins or figs, but only within very little quantities, if at all;
- Cashew nuts, pistachio and chestnuts.

Alcohol, for example: dry red and white wines and unsweetened spirits, but never when wanting to lose weight.

What foods should be completely avoided in the ketogenic diet?

- Avoid completely food rich in carbohydrates, meat made in a factory and treated foods.
- All granules, even whole meal of amaranth, sorghum, millet, corn, rye, wheat, oats, rice, buckwheat, germinated grains, white potatoes and quinoa. This includes every product made from grains, such as cookies, bread, pasta, pizza; sweeties similar to HFCS, table sugar, cakes, sugary puddings, soft-drinks and sugar;
- Factory-farmed fish and pork are rich in inflammatory omega 6 fatty acids, besides farmed fish might contain PCBs. Thus, avoid fish rich in mercury;
- Processed nourishment containing carrageenan, e.g. products from almond milk; MSG, e.g. some products with whey protein; sulphites, e.g. gelatin and dried fruits; BPAs or wheat gluten;
- Artificial sweeteners, for example: Saccharine, Equal, Splenda, sweeteners covering Aspartame or Sucralose;
- Refined fats, trans fats and oils, e.g. corn oil, sunflower, grape seed, safflower, soybean, cottonseed, margarine or canola;
- Low-fat, low or zero-carbohydrate products, say diet beverages, chewing mints and gums, as they are high with carbs or comprise gluten or artificial tastes;

- Milk, for tea and coffee replace it with a reasonable amount of cream. You might also have a little amount of uncooked milk, but just be wary of the added carbs;
- Alcoholic and sugary drinks, like beer, cocktails or sweet wine;
- Tropical fruit like tangerine, mango, grapes, pineapple, banana or papaya;
- Avoid fruit saps, instead drink shakes or smoothies, but in very small amounts. Juices are comparable to water with sugar, but smoothies hold fiber making it more filling. This likewise includes dried fruit, perhaps raisins or dates, but only when eaten in big quantities;
- Avoid wheat gluten, being usually utilized in foods low in carb;
- When giving up bread, try not to eat whatever part of it;
- Beware of BPA-lined containers. If likely, use obviously BPA-free packing, like crystal jars or create your own fixings of coconut milk, ketchup, ghee, or mayo. BPA is related to numerous negative wellbeing effects, similar to impaired thyroid functioning and tumors.

What can be an impeccable example of a ketogenic diet menu?

For breakfast:

- 4 ounces shredded beef mixed in spices,
- 1 ounce of sliced onion,
- 1 ounce of low-carb vegetables cooked in olive oil or butter,
- Unsweetened flavored tisane with hefty cream.

For lunch:

- 4 ounces oven-cooked halibut using sauce of dill butter,
- 1 cup cut cauliflower sautéed in olive oil or butter,
- 1 cup of salad greens peppered with blue cheese, besides a dressing of a tablespoon of full-fat vinaigrette,
- Unsweetened seasoned carbonated or plain water or any unsweetened beverage.

For dinner:

- 6 ounces baked pork chop with mashed garlic,
- 2 cups cut up cabbage cooked in buttered caraway,
- Salad greens using low-carb, high-fat dressing,
- Unsweetened flavored fresh water or any unsweetened liquid refreshment,

- Coffee with plentiful of cream.

How do you determine if you are in ketosis state or not?

The state of ketosis denotes that the physique has swapped from being dependent on carb for energy to use fats instead. This is clearly a wanted state for anyone aiming to drop extra pounds.

As you limit carbohydrates consumption and go with the nutritive fat, additional fats are metabolized and larger quantities of ketones are formed. The majority of cells inside your body, including those inside your brain become capable to tap ketones into energy with an adjustment phase of couple days.

Acetone, a variant of ketone, is not utilized by the body, thus is expelled as waste typically in the breath and urine. Conveniently, this makes it extremely simple to measure whether or not you are in ketosis.

Ketogenic breath:

Upon being bound into ketosis, selected people account for a change within the odor of their inhalation as an end result of the further released acetone. If you observe this occurring in the beginning of your nourishment change, it can be a wholesome sign that you are in the ketosis.

Ketones within urine:

The top accurate way to test ketosis is utilizing ketone urine examination bands, regularly alluding to Ketostix. These cheap testing bands are flawless and are made to instantly determine ketone intensities within your urine.

To do this, pass the examination end of the little paper band directly by your urine stream. Otherwise, amass urine inside a spotless parched vessel, and plunge the band inside. Dispose of whatever is extra and allow it to rest for a quarter of an hour.

If you are in ketosis, the band will alter color from its original shade. Liken the hue as instructed on the package to check if you hit your ketosis intensity. Deep purple color habitually defines progressive ketones level. Dimmer does not necessary mean better as plenty of people find low-to-medium ketosis levels to be excellent for direct fat deficit.

Beware that the ketone levels within the urine do not necessarily equal blood ketone intensities. The quantity of water you have inside your body can generate a huge difference regarding the intensity of ketones within your urine.

As time goes by, people adhering to ketogenic regimens have the tendency to gauge lower intensities of ketones within their urine, still remaining solidly within fat expend state. Now, a blood exam possibly is needed to precisely test ketosis, but these are significantly far expensive.

What is the difference between the ketogenic diet and Atkins diet?

Ketogenic nutrition is basically a diet that is within the shape of nutritional ketosis mainly. Most severe low-carb regimes limit daily carb intake of 50 grams or less.

On the other hand, an Atkins diet is a plan that includes starting in ketosis and continuing with ketosis till you succeed while losing a reasonable amount of body mass. This is called the induction phase.

After this, you slowly reintroduce carbohydrates and avoid junk carbs and sugars.

Conclusion

I hope that you have learned the real facts, the principles behind it, how it is beneficial to weight loss, the possible benefits and side effects, as well as the best practices to make your attempt to lose weight more successful.

Your next step is to apply everything you have learned from this book in your daily life. No matter how hectic your lifestyle it, take time to make use of the recipes, sample menus and food shopping tips presented in this book to and continually practice ketogenic diet.

Forget about starvation since ketogenic diet allows you to eat satisfyingly. Burn fat, lose weight fast by starting your new lifestyle today.

Good luck!

www.ingramcontent.com/pod-product-compliance
Lightning Source LLC
Chambersburg PA
CBHW071212280526
45787CB00002B/655